Thresholds

Thresholds

GLENNA COOK

Glenna Cook

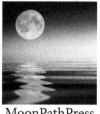

MoonPathPress

Poetry
ISBN 978-1-936657-28-5

Cover art: untitled acrylic, 30 inches x 22.5 inches,
1990s series, by the late Antje Kaiser, German born,
longtime resident of Tacoma.

Author photo: by Ken Cook

Design: Tonya Namura
using Cochin

MoonPath Press is dedicated to publishing the
finest poets of the U.S. Pacific Northwest.
MoonPath Press
PO Box 445
Tillamook, OR 97141

MoonPathPress@gmail.com
http://MoonPathPress.com

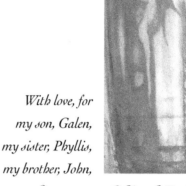

With love, for
my son, Galen,
my sister, Phyllis,
my brother, John,
and my parents, Sadie and Earl,
all who have crossed that final threshold

Contents

III Wake to December

Thresholds

I

Sister's Keeper

Contrary Is the Name My Parents Gave Me

Too young to remember, yet I remember:

Sitting in my spindly
wooden highchair,
I test its limits.

My foot against the kitchen table
tips it back.

More than once,
I push too far.

Easter Egg Hunt

At the signal, an army of children
lunges over the string fence
surrounding ten thousand
colored eggs planted on a battlefield of grass.

Grandfather lifts her over.
She holds tight the handle of her basket.

Grandfather shouts,
    Look, in front of you. There!
    No, there! Over there!

Faster legs dart in front of her,
swifter arms swoop up the plunder.

After the victors recede,
she stands among the litter of stepped-on eggs.

    Come, Grandfather tells her,
    It's time to go.

She steps over the sagging string,
holding out her empty basket,
a casualty of childhood's first war.

Bountiful Harvest

A pan of green beans in her lap,
a small girl sits on the floor.

She's surrounded by
legs clad in denim and work boots,
and legs beneath housedresses
wearing sensible shoes.

Above her floats a chorus of voices
from uncles, aunts, father, and mother.

They sit in a circle, snapping beans,
and telling stories that weave
together their everyday lives.

No one pays attention to the girl,
who listens.

She thinks,
I belong to them.
Contentment fills her belly.

Phyllis' Fate

A woman's body knows things.
Soon after the birth,
a doctor at Children's Hospital
confirmed my mother's pregnant fears.
Mongoloids, they called them, then.

> *She may never walk or feed herself,*
> *will never learn the things*
> *that normal children do.*
> *Best to place her in an institution.*

Numb silence on the bleak ride home,
doctor's words tearing her life.
Then, her husband reached across,
took her hand, and said,
> *She's ours.*
> *Let's keep her.*

Choice

Mother, if there had been tests,
and you had known,
would you still have chosen
to keep her?

I think you would have,
and considered yourself chosen, as well,
always looking for the good purpose
in what others might call catastrophe.

Now there are tests,
those who have an option,
but still some choose to learn
a new definition of perfection.

Fierce Love

Most people perceived you as flawed.
Mother saw you as blessing.

Her fierce love in your first months
brought you past pneumonia's peril.
She fed you goat milk, natural vitamins.
Mrs. Mann massaged you
with her miracle hands.
You thrived.

Rather than hide you in the shadows,
she placed you at the heart of things —
center stage.

At church gatherings, school carnivals,
there you'd be, perched on her lap,
or atop Father's shoulders,
curious gaze taking in a world
difficult for you to comprehend,
yet, one where she'd always
make a place for you.

Ritual

Every morning the same,
the four of us at breakfast.
Father hears you from the bedroom,
carries you out, a stinky bundle
wrapped in soaked, flannel blanket.

He jokes,
> *Look what I found!*
> *She must have fallen in a river.*

I think,
> *That's not funny*
> *   not funny*
> *   not funny.*

Your dark eyes peer out,
pink cheeks,
innocent smile.

Mother reaches to take you
into her arms.

I think,
> *How can they love her*
> *   love her*
> *   love her,*

> *so much?*

1940: Riding with Uncle George at Four Years Old

I point to the long, metal stick
attached to the floor
that he keeps moving
around with his hand,
and say, what's that?

He says, it's a gear shift,
and I say, what's it for?

And he says, it changes
the gears from one to another.

And I say, what's a gear?

And he says, it's what makes
the car move —
low gears for going slow,
high gears for going fast.

And I say, oh,
not understanding everything,
but feeling much smarter.

Here's what really happens:

I point to the funny stick
coming out of the floor,
and say, what's that?

And he says, it's just
something to make little girls
ask questions.

And I say
nothing more.

Ethel, 1886 to 1931

As for mortals, their days are as grass:
they flourish like a flower of the field;
for the wind passes over it, and it is gone;
and its place knows it no more.
                                        Psalm 103

My grandmother died before I was born.
Breast cancer took her, at age forty-five.

Those, now gone, who knew her,
said she was gentle and generous,
had a quirky sense of humor.

She married young,
bore seven children,
dragged them from town to town,
as her husband followed carpentry jobs.
The houses they lived in were shabby.
She scoured them with vengeance.

She herded her family to church on Sundays,
sewed quilts at the women's mission group,
fed hungry hoboes who knocked at her door.

She loved to rest on the porch,
a pan of apples on her lap
to peel and parcel to her children,
as she sang them sad songs:

Oh don't you remember, a long time ago,
those two little babes, their names I don't know,
were stolen away, one bright summer day,
and lost in the woods, so I heard people say . . .

A small, serious woman,
dressed in somber clothes,
looks out from the only photograph
I own of her.

Her eyes do not expect too much.

This Poem Is for You, Johnny

It was her or you.
Father had to choose her.

In the days before ultra-sound,
routine C-sections,
your size did you in —
ten-pound Titan,
wrenched from Mother's tiny body.

She held you in her arms,
a perfectly beautiful baby boy.
It had to be her.

If you had lived,
you would have been
a motherless child,
raised by a broken father.

I wouldn't be here,
nor would our sister and brother.
We rode in on the wave
of your passing.

You would be over eighty, now,
with stories to tell.

Instead, there's a small marker
at the cemetery.

I'm writing this poem for you,
Johnny, to say I wish
you both could have lived.

Stepping Stone

Mother irons father's Sunday
dress shirt while you, Phyllis,
perch at her feet,
crouching under the board.

I ask Mother why you can't
walk and talk
like other kids your age.

This is the moment
she hands me the heavy weight
of your condition,
sets upon my slumped shoulders
my duty as your sister.

This is the moment
I begin to understand
why you take up so much space
that used to be mine.

Property Lines

Fishing poles in hand,
we kids clambered through brush
and over fallen logs,
following the meandering creek
in pursuit of six-inch rainbows.

Scratched by devil's club,
stung by nettles,
wet and muddy,
we didn't think about boundaries
and didn't care who lived in
the out-of-sight houses
on top of the gully.

But when old Mr. Anderson logged-off
the back of his place,
and the liberated blackberries
thrived over the stumps,
he made his property off-limits to us.

The Anderson clan filled
bucket after bucket,
and sold them in town,
ten dollars a gallon.

We thought it unfair.
Didn't woods and blackberries
belong to everyone?

Doing It in the Third Grade

I

Miss Barton's class, a worksheet
of addition on my desk.

September sun warms
through the window,
calls me outside.

Shadows of leaves
flicker across my paper.
I smell trees.

I smell the smooth,
skinny-trunked trees
my brother taught me
to shinny up.
> *Place your hands high, your feet
> around the trunk, push-pull up, and repeat.*

I shinny high,
press my body against the trunk
to hold me, and, oh, a sweetness.

A sweetness in my body,
down there,
an electric sweetness.

My brother slides down his tree,
but I stay high
to feel the sweetness.

September sun warms my body,
moves me in my seat,
moves me back and forth.

I move softly, slowly,
so no one will notice.

Morris, in the desk next to mine
works on his sums.

I press down, swaying
until the sweetness returns,
the sweetness in my body.

Suddenly, I shudder.

Morris' head jerks up,
our eyes meet.

II

I keep doing it.
I don't want to,
but every day
sitting so long in my seat,
a tightness in my body
pushes in on me until
I think I will shatter,
and then I do it.

Miss Barton knows
and punishes me,
keeps me after school.

She says my answers are wrong,
even though I know
they are right.
She says, do them again.

The paper has holes from erasing.
I have tried every answer.

She leaves the room,
but I see her peek in.
She wants to know if I'm doing it.

III

Betty Ann said she tried
what I do
at home.
She liked it.

She became my friend.

But the next day,
her mother told her
it was bad.

She's not my friend, anymore.

IV

Does my mother know?

Does my father know?

Does Miss Barton tell them
I do it?

No one talks to me about it.

No one tells me it's wrong.

No one tells me to stop.

V

I want it to be my secret
even though I know
everyone knows
I do it.

A World of Your Own

Phyllis, you talk to yourself,
a characteristic of Down syndrome.
I can never hear the words
of your conversations,
low tones, answered in whispers.
You confide, laugh, affectionately chide,
as good friends do.

When I was four, and you, a baby,
our family moved out of town.
No other kids lived in our neighborhood.
Our brother in school,
Mother busy with housework and you,
I chose my own imaginary playmates
to keep away the loneliness.

But, as I grew, this circle of friends
(scorned by some adults)
became inaccessible.

For you, though, a diaphanous fabric
still flutters between reality and fantasy,
allowing you to escape at will
into an enviable secret world of your own.

The Top Bunk

You, Brother, being oldest, wanted it,
but Mother said you might fall
if you sleep-walked, again.

I like to think
she knew
I needed it more than you.

I like to think she knew
I would lie awake at night,
my head at the foot of my bed
by the open window,
listen to the frogs creak
from the marsh,
watching meteors streak across
the black August sky.

I like to think she knew
I would wake up in grayness
to the mournful cry
of fog horns from the bay
and the sparkle of spider webs
strung between dry corn stalks.

I like to think she knew
the cool breeze that blew
across me
washed away
my loneliness.

New Girl

Only two mornings you ride my school bus.
You glide, eyes down, past silence and sullen looks.

I don't know why you sit beside me,
except that you see I am also alone.

The second day, I don't leave any room.
You sit across the aisle from me.

The year is 1945. Our town is as white
as the sleet that assails the bus window.

You have just skinned your knee.
I have never seen blood on black skin before.

The school bus quivers on the icy street.
A ruby glistens on smooth, dark satin.

The Swing

I

The amazing thing was not the swing,
but my father, balanced like a cat,
or the logger he used to be,
spurring up a spar tree,
his body a steel spring.

We craned our necks to see him hoist,
with help of block and tackle,
a peeled alder, newly cut,
to span the space between
the sturdy crotches
of two ancient maples.

A swing so tall,
its ropes so thick and heavy—
it could have held an elephant.

He laughed to see his achievement.

No amount of pumping could ever
coax a good momentum out of it.

II

A neighbor boy, older than me,
pushed me on that swing.

He flipped my dress
and promised to show me how
babies are made.

I lied, said I knew,
and ran home to tell my mother.

Next day, I saw him on our front step,
getting a long talk from my father.

That boy never came near me again.

In the Middle

My big brother,
bright, shining star,
born after the death
of the first son,
can do no wrong.

My little sister,
sweet darling,
born with Down syndrome,
can do little right.
Still, everything she does
amazes them.

By myself,
I learn to ride a boy's bike,
memorize times tables,
earn stars on teacher's chart.
It doesn't matter.

I'm supposed to understand,
the oldest, and a boy,
has first place.

I'm supposed to understand,
sister's special needs mean
no time for mine.

I'm supposed to know,
smart, strong and normal,
I can make it on my own.

My Sister's Keeper

I couldn't accept her abnormalities,
bore them strapped to my back.

God knows I tried to make her right.
When she didn't walk by two,
I held her hands above her head,
guiding her unsure steps until she could.

For me, not her,
I prodded her toward normality.
   Stop slurping your soup.
   Keep your tongue in your mouth.

At every family picnic, she'd wander away.
We'd all fan out to find her —
once, eating ice cream with a group of strangers,
once, crouched at the end of a diving board,
once, she fell off a slide and broke her collar bone.

Sometimes, I took her with me
to my friend's house.
Time to come home,
she'd plant herself,
limp as an oyster.
I'd fuss and rant,
try to lift her by her flaccid arms.
My friend's mother would smile and say,
   Just start walking. She'll come.
She would, like a bear cub
following its mama.
She'd come off as the smart one,
and I, the cranky oppressor.

Mother said that taking care
of my sister
would make me a better person.
I never once believed her.

Because I was talking

trying to be heard
in the usual breakfast confusion,
Mother didn't see you, Phyllis,
reach for fresh-poured coffee.

Because my talking distracted Mother,
your screams followed me to school,
where I didn't hear teacher call on me,
missed spelling words that I knew.

I bought candy raspberry vines for you,
spending my week's allowance.

Because, Mother says
children with Down syndrome
don't hurt as long as normal children do,
you stopped crying,
even before the doctor dressed
the peeled, red burn on your thigh.

That's why you're content
on Mother's lap
when I come home
and give you a raspberry vine.

And that's why I am still hurting.

They Used to Be My Toys

Those little black garters
with white stripes
slithered over backyard grass.

I'd grab them by the tail,
hold them in my hands
until I grew
tired of them,
or merciful.
Then, I'd let them go.

At twelve, I picked one up
to show my cousins
how silly it was to be fearful.
>   *See*, I taunted,
>   *there is no reason to be afraid.*

The creature dangling
from my fingers
stiffened,
crooked its sinuous body
and looked at me,
froze me
with its lidless eyes.
>   *Now I have the power,*
>   it seemed to say.

I screamed,
and flung it away.

The Day I Teach My Sister to Open a Door

Again, she has imprisoned herself
in the bedroom,
rousing me from my book.

She pounds the door and sounds
her guttural cry
for someone to release her.

No one, except me,
seems to mind these vexations.
My flung book lies open on the floor.

When I enter the bedroom
and slam the door,
she shrinks like a cornered rabbit.

I squeeze her hand
around the doorknob,
jerk her body
in relentless motion:
    turn, pull, open, shut,
    turn, pull, open, shut.

Lesson over,
she opens the door,
remains in its threshold,
laughing.

Looking Back on the Face of War

At school,
they take our fingerprints.
We practice air-raid drills,
paste savings stamps,
save tin-foil off gum wrappers,
stamp cans flat.

World War II is a game.

In the woods, we play war,
wake each day to rumble
of guns from the fort,
identify our fighter planes
flying overhead,
climb aboard Navy ships
docked in our port.

On cozy nights,
behind darkened windows,
we huddle by our radio
to hear news of distant battles,
and Uncle George sends horned toads
from an Army camp in Texas.
We feed them flies, but they die.

A newsreel at the movies shows
snow falling on broken shells of houses,
men throwing logs into the back of a truck.

The camera zooms in,
reveals not wood,
but a girl my age,

one leg crooked at the knee —
solid ice in sleep position.

I see the face of war,
eyelids frozen open.

Phyllis at the Birthday Party

I

It's your first time on the bus.
I lift you onto the seat.
You gape at other passengers,
who steal glances.

As we get off,
you stumble,
dangle from my hand
like a marionette.

I kneel down,
look you over,
all dressed up for the party,
ribbon in your hair, new dress.

For the first time,
I see how beautiful you are,
your face, a moon
reflected on a placid sea.

I crush your doll-body
to my skinny chest.

When I release you,
a ripple crosses your brow.
You swallow.

II

After the party,
when our aunt tells you
to pick up the wrapping paper
you've strewn over the lawn,
I fly into a rage.
        She can't help it!
I storm around,
gathering the garbage.

Going Fishing with My Dad and Brother

I'd forget, sometimes,
how it was the last time,
and beg to go with them again.

Early next morning,
I'd be jostled from sleep,
rushed through breakfast,
left to finish
while they loaded
tackle and boat.

They'd wait, impatient
for me to get into the truck.

At the lake dock, they'd launch,
and with me in the stern,
take off rowing.

They'd talk softly
between themselves,
not let me talk at all.

    You'll scare the fish, they said.

All morning long,
they'd feed worms onto hooks,
row back and forth,
back and forth,
catch an occasional fish.

Every bite they got meant
another pass, and another cast,

until I was hungry, cold, bored
and had to pee.

You insisted on coming.

Smelly fish flopped
in the bottom of the boat.
Patterns of color swirled
in the water going by,
an endless, slow motion movie.

Horror Movie

The day after my sister and I
saw the up-raised hand
of Ricardo Montalbán sink slowly
into quicksand,
she developed Bell's palsy.

Mother scolded me for taking her
to a horror movie.
At twelve, I didn't know
the second feature was
always frightening.

Her lopsided expression for months,
until she got her real face back,
was my punishment.

Phyllis, with her penguin walk,
flat features,
and odd way of talking,
because of me,
had to wear that eerie,
twisted smile.

Old Mrs. Ornette

When I was eight, my mother made me walk the half-mile down our country road to buy eggs from old Mrs. Ornette. More than her black dog that hounded my heels, or her hissing geese that spread their ornery wings, it was Mrs. Ornette, herself, who filled me with dread. Hushed and sinister, she loomed like a giant loaf of white bread, her head an unbaked dinner roll with two raisins stuck in for eyes, a white bun coiled on top. She belonged to one of those churches that teaches that everything pleasant is sin.

When she opened the screen door to hand me the eggs and take my thirty-five cents, I could smell the Hell and Brimstone she exhaled.

Old *Mr.* Ornette, raucous and irreverent, as she was quiet and pious, was her cross to bear, but then he died.

Their granddaughter, Marie, my age, lived with her. I tried to be friends, but her mind always skittered off, maybe chasing after her parents, who were who knows where?

Soon after the old man died, I sat on the stoop of a tool shed with Marie and her cousin, Clyde. She told me how once the two of them had peeked through the window of that shed, saw Grandpa with three teen-aged girls, one of them Clyde's sister. Clyde stopped her story with a look. What was left unsaid hovered over us, so I hurried home before it blocked out the sun, as I blocked out the memory.

Recently, it came to mind again, and I wondered, was Mrs. Ornette really so mean, or just plain miserable?

The last I time I saw Marie, she wore a black suit that fit nicely over her curvaceous figure. She told me she was friends with a whole minor-league baseball team.

Word Keeper

I'm sorry
about my words.
I try to keep them in
behind their white picket fence,
but they get out when I least expect it.
Just when I think I have them tamed
and trained to stay where they belong,
they squirm under or jump over the gate,
or escape when I forget to close it.
Then, they run and there's just no stopping them.
I hope they haven't been a nuisance,
or caused you any harm.
I'll do what I can to
keep them in, but
I can't promise
they won't
get out
again.

Windstorm

We stand at the window
watching trees fall
                          one
        by one
tall firs and hemlocks
                  crashing
in random order
        like pick-up sticks
their root systems
                turning up as walls
my brother and I will climb
        next day
to survey the damage

Taunting the Storm

After days and days
of dry summer heat,
the sky went crazy,
exploding in rapid bursts
from every direction,
brilliant razzle-dazzle light.

I ran out in my nightgown,
wild and reckless,
my youthful intrepidness
taunting the storm.

The heavy rain roared like a cataract,
streamed down my body,
while all around me
the air sizzled.

Sheets of electric neon flashed
on and off, on and off,
blue, magenta, orange, white.

My jubilant screams
joined the rolling timpani.

Boom! Rumble! Boom!

I spread my arms,
lifted my face to the pelting rain,
and danced, whirling and jumping,
my soul surrendered to the elements.
I was sixteen.

Oh, to be sixteen once more.

To Irene

Walking down Olympia's Capitol Way,
from the cold stadium
where our high school team
had just won their football game,
we stopped at the Dairy Queen
and bought vanilla ice cream cones,
a silly thing to do on a snowy day.

We laughed at ourselves,
though ice cream had never
tasted so delicious.

We were so close, that day,
happy in our own world
that required nothing of us,
beyond being who we were.

Where did careless winds,
over thoughtless time
blow that happiness,
that bond of friendship?

Stars landed on your black
and my brown hair.
Our laughter pealed like bells.
Our breath froze in the cold, pure air.

Sex in the Fifties

Good girls didn't have sex.

We wondered why Stella
withdrew from us,
the last month of ninth grade.
Every day, she wore the same
loose shirt, and then she didn't
show up for tenth.

In eleventh grade,
beautiful blonde Mona,
with her neat little body,
didn't almost die
from using a coat hanger.
She had a ruptured appendix.

And even those of us
who squeaked by
with precious membrane
still intact on her wedding day,
could feel our parents' anxious
eyes upon us,
until enough childless months
had passed.

Candle Lighter

Mother wanted to know if
you were going to be in my wedding.
Her sour expression accused me.

Vexed, I said you'd be a candle lighter.

Now, as I wait for Father
to walk me down the aisle,
I watch you through a crack in the door.

You float along the sanctuary
lighting candles in each window,
working your way to
the candelabra near the altar.

You wear an airy dress of lavender organdy,
ribbon around your dark-brown hair,
white Mary-Jane's.

I can almost see your wings.

Face shining with devotion,
illuminating the room as you move along,
you raise the light above you.

Down Syndrome and Eros

Marriage, not in your future,
Phyllis, you will never have
a lover, except for George,
a yard of white and black
striped pillow-ticking,
filled with goose-down,
held in your arms at night,
or laid between your thighs.

Who's to say
your whispered exchanges
and heart-felt sighs
are not as meaningful
as anything we've experienced
in our connubial beds?

Who's to say the passions you know
with this imaginary person,
do not come close
to those the rest of us seek
in our quest for perfect love?

II

Two Dreams

Crustaceans

This man who towers above her
and drills her with his voice,
as a moon snail drills with acid
through oyster shells,
is not his true self.

Nor is her true self
this passive blob of jelly,
silent and defenseless,
unable to speak the apology
he demands,
or think of any word
that would make a difference.

Out the window,
crustacean-covered rocks line the shore.
They once knew their true selves.

Before barnacles and limpets attached,
waves washed smooth surfaces,
sun cast clean shadows upon the sand.

When this argument is over,
she'll retreat to a quiet place
to heal her injury.

He'll come back,
more sorrowful than sorry,
and want her to heal him, too.

All the while he is shouting,
she is thinking about crustaceans.

Morning Message from the Sea

Mist blurs the horizon line, closes in,
keeps out the world beyond.

Quicksilver waves heave and dip,
crest and slide across the sand to meet me.

I have come to say goodbye,
my tears flowing.

Foam caresses my ankles.
Something in me whispers —

> *Be glad for what is in your life.*
> *It is enough.*

I pocket a small, white shell
and walk back home.

If I Needed Proof

This morning,
as a flame-colored sky
silhouettes
the bare-limbed cherry tree,
you could stop me
from going.

One word from you,
and I would beg
my heart to cease
its wandering.

Or you could come with me.

I would try to match my pace,
my taste to yours,
though we both know
that has never worked before.

If I needed proof
you still love me,
it would be in the way
you let me go—
still holding fast
your end of my tether,
so when I've seen enough,
I come safely home
to the familiar
continent of your embrace.

And just now,
the slanted rays
of winter sun

illumine,
on the table between us,
the scarlet tips
of imported tulips.

Two Dreams

Last night, after our quarrel,
you slept poorly,
dreamed you bought
two Volkswagen Passats
and drove them into our bedroom.

I slept well, and dreamed I made
two pots of Japanese vegetable soup,
ladled it into earthenware bowls,
and served people gathered at our house.

Sharing our dreams this morning,
I feel the insistent crowding of the cars,
and wonder if you feel
the nurturing warmth of the soup.

My Father Died at Eighty-Eight

That day, he picked bluebells
and made love to my mother.

His heart gave out from such foolishness.

A man plans differently

than a woman for a journey.
He sees where he is going,
finds the shortest route
to get there and return,
takes two changes of clothes,
a little bag of toiletries.
Money.

A woman looks
at what is being left behind,
cleans her house
for coming home to,
tells the people in her life
where she's going,
when she'll be back.
Someone must be found
to tend her plants
and care for her cat.
She packs three sets of clothes
for every change of weather,
bakes nut bread
to eat along the way.

When a woman takes a trip to London

she must first unweave
from her daily fabric,
prepare ahead for needs
of all who depend on her,
tell those who expect her
at certain times
to be at certain places
that she won't.

It's a bit like dying.

She prepares herself, too —
bargains with guilt
as she shelves responsibility,
gathers courage to face
the unknown of traveling alone.

To justify the trip,
she vows to make the most of it.
It can't be just a respite,
a well-deserved vacation.
It has to have a purpose,
as perhaps, a call from God.

When she has finally cleared
the hurdles, she finds
herself airborne,
having checked her baggage
with a mix of relief to be rid of it
and fear she will never see it again.

She looks down on where she has been,
perceives the weaving of the threads —

the lives she touches,
her home, her duties, her art —
not as unrelated strands,
but as a whole piece.

From this distance, she knows
that her life below is happy.
She smiles as the distance grows.

I wonder who will be next?

Mother remarked,
on one of our slow rides
to the cemetery in a black limousine.

This time,
it was Uncle Bill.

They are all gone, now,
plucked one-by-one,
like berries from a bush
by a hungry bird.

Now, it is *my* generation
who waits,
so much overripe fruit,
dangling.

The Waiting Room

I bring something to read or write,
anything to pass the time.

Mother simply waits,
accustomed to days that dawdle
their progress toward dark,
or nights whose sleepless hours
drag in the morning.

She waits for her bath,
for mealtimes,
for her chair
to be pushed to the table,
for eye drops, pills,
and a kiss at bedtime.

Restless, I pace,
stopping to watch fish
clean the aquarium glass
with their busy snouts.

I too swim in a sea
of perpetual motion.

Unlike fish,
who have no sense of future,
I cannot wait —
yet I wait —
for the waiting to be over.

Mother Stands on the Threshold

A stroke crept into your brain
in the dark hours of morning,
found where you store your words,
jumbled them,
threw your most precious to the winds —
names of your children,
your dead husband.

The doctor said
you wouldn't last three months.
Three years later,
you say you are ready,
but that strength within you,
the same strength that marshaled order
for those around you,
works against your will to go.

You straighten, precisely,
the contents of your dresser drawers,
refuse to go out with your bra-straps showing,
or to sit in the lobby drowsing your days.
And when you roll your walker down the hall,
you strive to stand erect.

Though you insist we take you
to church on Sunday,
you sleep through the service,
tell me with gestures and faltering words,
that you no longer find God there.

Instead, he comes in the night,
lifts you out of your body,

and just when you think
you are going home,
brings you back by morning.

You stand on the threshold,
content to cross over,
but making sure that all things
are in their right places
on this side before you go.

The Peeler

I stand, impatient, Mother,
watching you peel peaches.
You slash and gouge,
remove the unripe skin
in thick and wasteful slices.
You tremble in your haste
and grunt with the effort.

I am reminded of being wakened
from childhood summer dreams,
to join you in your steamy kitchen
where I helped preserve
the golden fruit,
picked the day before
at its peak of sweetness.

No waste then.
Emerging from their bath
of scalding water,
their peels slipped off clean
in our fingers,
and my small hand fit them,
halved,
into their jars
like flower petals upside down.

Just so,
or you made me
do them over.

I hate the way
you are peeling now,

because I'm afraid
I shall be like you someday,
waking my daughter at six a.m.
to tell her in my stroke-broken speech
that I dreamed of peaches last night,
and I fear the season might pass
before I taste one.

I Confess

I wanted you to die.

The last time you wavered,
I had hoped you would move
with graceful and courageous step
through that luminous door.

In the face of its bright promise,
why feel obliged to stay
in this grim twilight,
sucking dwindled pleasures dry
from the sagging tit of old age?

I sit with you in this place
that bears within its dark smells
the fact of our mortality.

I confess that I know nothing.

You hold me in the spell
of your clear-eyed gaze,
your incongruous smile.

You have awakened
from dreams of wheat fields
and maple trees.

Children pass by
like rustling leaves.

Slow Journey

Nothing prepared her
to care for her mother.

She hadn't known to practice
moving in slow motion.

When Time trapped her
in its viscous flow,
she strained her limbs
against the density,
saw her life suspended
in congealing globs of duty.

She cried:
When I escape from this,
will my dreams still be waiting?

Time answered
Only one dream matters —
the one too close to see —
an elegant dance in rhythm with me.

Haydn's Quartet in F Major

Two centuries ago,
some ancestors
whose names I don't know,
grew cotton and flax,
spun it into thread,
then wove a bedspread in simple
Pennsylvania Dutch design —
rose-colored flowers,
Sunday-blue leaves,
on cream background.

I wish I had asked for more stories.
Those who would tell them are gone.
I stand between fragments
and the encroaching future,
listening to a compact disc
play Haydn's three-century-old
Quartet in F Major.

I fold the bedspread — insect-chewed
in spots, unraveling on the edges,
and place it in the homemade chest
my mother had kept in her kitchen
for tea towels and tablecloths.

Through my open window,
the call of finches.

Sometimes Away: A Villanelle

You need from me what I cannot give,
my mind, my choice, my inner space.
I give you what I can, a single love.

You want togetherness—hand in glove,
and knock on the door of my private place.
You need from me what I cannot give.

A flower needs the sun to thrive.
From you, my son, I sometimes turn my face.
I give you what I can, a single love.

What I withhold, I ask you to forgive.
I cannot be a flower in a vase.
You need from me what I cannot give.

Sometimes, away from you, I move,
and yet, I need you as home base.
I give you what I can, a single love.

For me, your love is like that from above,
holding my limitations in your embrace.
You need from me what I cannot give.
I give you what I can, a single love.

Montana Mountains

Your solid presence hems me in
and blocks from view
the brilliant hues of red and gold,
cast low in the sky at sunrise and sunset.

Your forbidding slopes,
home to cougar, bear, and wolf,
are safe from my approach.

Earth lifted up by tectonic heaves,
your ancient history gives
little consolation.

We will all disappear
and you will still be here.

Montana Night Message

Every night,
I step outside to view the stars.

When moonshine dims the stars,
I gaze at the moon.

When clouds cover moon and stars,
I listen to the sigh of wind as it swishes
through fir, pine, and tamarack trees.
It touches my face with cool fingers.

The night humbles me.
Stars, moon, wind,
and towering trees,
make me feel small.

What am I among
this grandeur of the universe?

I am here to bear
the privilege of awareness.

Yes, this world could do without me,
yet, I matter.

Grass Roots Revolution

I killed a thistle today,
the most beautiful plant in my garden,
a crocheted doily of gray-green
leaves, spread out in perfect symmetry.

If I had left it, a three-foot stalk
would have grown from its center,
with branches of needle-tipped leaves
and prickly heads crowned in purple,
which soon would turn white and fly
silk parachutes in the wind.

And that's not even to say
how it would attract goldfinches,
those black and yellow songbirds,
rarely seen in the city where
thistles are not allowed to grow.

I wish I could have let my thistle grow,
and all the other so-called weeds in my yard:
dandelion, bindweed, buttercup and clover.

I wouldn't mow my lawn,
and let the tall grass
invite garter snakes and field mice,
a covey of quail, some rabbits.

I'd have my own eco-system
on this little plot.

My neighbors would think this unsightly,
complain when seeds blew

through the chain-link
into their medicated yards.

And their cats, tired of dried pellets,
might eat the little birds and animals.

An urban lot is no place for paradise.

So I destroyed my thistle,
before it could start a revolution.

And I pulled out all the other weeds.
My yard looks conforming and neat.

Those splendid goldfinches must fly
somewhere else to nest.

I take comfort in knowing that,
try as I might,
the weeds will keep coming back.

It would be impossible
to eliminate all the deep-rooted
thistles on this planet.

Urban Capitalists

Squirrels run spirals up and down my trees,
play tag with privileged nonchalance.

Throughout autumn months,
fat and sleek
in their impeccable gray suits,
they have acquired
more, more, more,
until their storehouses are full,
and they bury nuts in the ground.

If they forget where they put
their investments,
their nose for profit will sniff
them out.

Or else, nuts forgotten
will grow into trees —
possibilities for future gain —
a trickle-down benefit for the forest,
an irritating nuisance in a city yard.

Deep in their memories,
they must have a lean year,
when drought,
then early deep-freeze
made for scarce pickings,
when they survived
by robbing bird feeders.

Right now, a sharp-eyed sentinel,
perched on a high branch,

flags his plumy tail
and warns in a loud
chirr, chirr, chirr,
the cat slouching under the juniper.

Truce

On this acre of land in Montana
I use a pickax to pry sticks
and roots from topsoil scraped aside
to make room for our new home.
I work to recover compost
left by trees now cut down.
Foreign, noxious weeds—
knapweed, ox eye, hawk eye, and tansy—
quickly invade
the clay laid bare by the dozer.

A line of black ants passes,
displaced refugees,
plodding single-file
across barren earth
toward distant green.

> *If you don't mess with me*, I say,
> *I won't mess with you.*

Once, when we lived in Tacoma,
my husband waged war
against squirrels
that chewed on our house,
built nests inside the eves.
He attacked them with his pellet gun.
The first gulf war had just begun.

> *Stop!* I said.
> *There has been enough bloodshed.*

I prayed for the squirrels,
and called a truce.

For my sake, he put away his gun.
Believe it or not,
the squirrels left us alone
for a few years,
then my husband
saw one go into the eves again.

One shot through the head.
It froze, then toppled, rigid and dead.

Fully aware that I am
the foreign invader,
and that my big nest displaces
a long-established order,
I offer a truce to all creatures who
come to this acre in Montana —

> bears who invade my garbage can,
> cougars looking for neighborhood cats,
> deer who devour my tomatoes,
> return to a place that once was theirs.

St. Regis, Montana, New Year's Eve 2009

I'm outside looking for the Blue Moon,
second full moon of a month.

Nineteen-eighty-nine was the last time
one appeared on New Year's Eve.

Next time, twenty-twenty-eight,
and also a total lunar eclipse.

I hope I'm alive to see it.

I wait in the darkness, my eyes
pointing to the place the moon should be.

Tall firs stand sentinel,
silent in the windless, cold air.

It begins to snow and I'm about to
go inside, when the clouds open.

Through a veil, she gazes down at me.
A soft aura surrounds her beautiful face.

A few seconds, then the clouds close.
Once in a blue moon, an impossible gift.

This time, I was ready.

Separate Courses

I go my own way,
husband, children, career,
seldom thinking of you, Phyllis.

A carefree teen,
you breeze your blue Schwinn
through the neighborhood,
ride your slow horse, Lucky,
charge the neighbor kids ten cents
for a turn around the yard,

In your room, you listen
to Lawrence Welk and Ernie Ford,
rock to Elvis, your greatest love.

You are the first person
with Down syndrome
hired by the State of Washington.

For nineteen years, you film
documents onto microfiche.

We continue our separate courses,
until Father's death
makes me your legal guardian,
and Mother's stroke
leaves you solely in my care.

At the senior home,
where you live alone,
I show you how to do laundry,
help you buy groceries,
a new jacket when your zipper breaks,

take you to doctor, dentist, beauty salon,
see you have money for the pop machine.

You know a phone call will bring me.
    Glenna, I'm sorry, I made a mess.

Three a.m., thirty miles on the freeway.
I clean you up and take your temperature.
I don't mind.
You are not the burden I expected.

For the next nine years,
until your death,
I want only to protect you.

Liberation

My sister Phyllis is going to
Morningside's first dance.
As she dons her black polyester slacks
and silky, cerise polyester shirt,
her face glows with anticipation.

The music is loud
and all the specially challenged,
even those in wheelchairs,
are rocking and rolling,
swinging and swaying,
clapping and stomping,
twirling and burning up the floor.

They dance faces up, eyes closed, voices raised
as they sing along with the music —
Dionysius' happy people.

Don't think for a minute they don't know
they are different.

They've seen a life-time of stares,
carefully averted eyes,
condescending friendliness.

But tonight, it's safe to be different.
Tonight, normal is not normal
and there is a place
in this world for them,
right here with Elvis, the Beatles,
Jeremiah Bullfrog, Mack the Knife,
and *Y.-M.-C.-A.*

The Apartment

I decide it's time you live
in your own apartment, Phyllis,
and find a studio close to your work.

Together, we shop for all you need,
bought with your own money.
What fun to open boxes,
put everything away.

A woman comes once-a-week,
helps with shopping and meals.
You keep the apartment clean,
stay with Mother on weekends.

At a grocery store nearby,
you spot a Budweiser sign.
Beer! you say,
with a gleam in your eye.
I say, *If there is beer,*
there will be no apartment.

Phyllis' Petty Crime

Pop is your problem.
Diet Pepsi, preferably.
We give you money
for the vending machine.

You spend it all,
and it's never enough.

We send three cans
in your backpack.
It's never enough.

You devise ways to get it.
Who knew Down syndrome
could be so creative?

You panhandle in the office lobby,
swipe pop from the fridge,
jostle coats on the rack
for the jingle of coins,
pilfer the coffee fund,
steal from Mother's purse.

You Zerox copies of a dollar bill
and use them in the vending machine.
The F.B.I. questions you,
then lets you go.

We talk to you, repeatedly.
You promise, never again.

You are the raccoon that steals
into our garden and eats our corn.
So pesky and persistent,
so innocent and cute,
an unmasked bandit
we really don't want to punish.

Lady of the Manor

My sister invites her office
for lunch at her senior home.

In a panic, I begin the arrangements:
negotiate a date with her boss,
plan a menu with the kitchen staff,
shop with Phyllis for decorations.

When the day arrives,
they all carpool across town.

The staff treat Phyllis
as Lady of the Manor,
serve lunch at her gala event.

After her guests have eaten,
she takes them to her apartment,
neat and shining with Christmas color.
This is my couch, this is my TV,
    this is my table, this is my bed . . .
She lists each item with pride, as if to say,
    I have a life, like you.

The Light Begins to Dim

Shadows steal your memory, Phyllis,
play tricks with your sense of time.

Three times within five minutes,
as I drive you in my car,
you ask how I am doing.
> I say, *I'm doing fine.*
> You say, *That's good.*

No longer punctual for work,
you arrive an hour early one day,
two hours late the next.

I fear I'm losing you.
Are you afraid of losing me?

For two solid weeks before Thanksgiving,
you called me almost every morning.
Your bags were packed,
why wasn't I there to pick you up?

And then, last night,
standing outside your senior home,
drenched in your work clothes,
shivering in the January rain,
you thought it was morning,
and had waited hours in the dark,
for a bus that didn't come.

Your working days are over.

As the light begins to dim,
I'm bringing you home
to live with me.

Evening Ritual with Phyllis

Every day you live with us,
I wash the dishes, you dry,
my husband, Ken, puts away.
Among the clatter,
you two banter back and forth.

He says, with mock impatience,
   Hurry up. You're too slow.
And you, pretending to be offended, say,
   Now, now,
        or,
   Watch it, Bub,
        or,
   You better watch your P.U.D.'s.

This, until the last dish is put away,
and you have carefully hung
the damp towel on its rack.

One night, in a rush to go to a movie,
we send you to the bathroom to get ready.
You come out, see Ken drying
and putting away.

You lean against the wall
and watch, your face downcast.

   Phyllis, what's the matter?
I ask.

You answer with stifled sob,
   He's taken my job.

Phyllis: Beginning of the End

I

On your fifty-ninth birthday,
Ken and I treat you
to your favorite dinner:

Big Mac with French fries,
a large diet Coke.

Then, to see The Straight Story,
about a man who drives
a riding lawnmower
three hundred miles
to see his brother,
estranged and ill from a stroke.

When the lights come on,
you're smiling.

Arms linked with Ken and me,
you walk between us,
out of the theater, to the car,
smiling, smiling, smiling.

II

Soon after your birthday,
you have a stroke.

It takes away your balance,
puts you in the nursing home,

the same one where Mother lives,
and it's bliss for her to have you there.

With her one good foot,
she paddles her wheelchair
down to your room,
to mother you, again.

You seem *not* to want her fuss.
You'd rather come
home with us.

III

The occupational therapist explains
all the things we'd need to do
to make it safe for you
to live with us.

With Mother in the nursing home,
this extra care of you
would be three hundred miles
too much.

I stand at the door
of your new room,
at the assisted care facility,
preparing to leave you here.

As I say goodbye,
you, hunched in a chair,
plush raccoon hugged to your chest,
won't look at me.

IV

You've stopped the daily packing
of your bags
for coming home.

Instead, you join in the activities,
cart dozens of *National Geographics*
to your room.

At breakfast, you say
to your stubborn tablemate,
> *If you take your pills, Rosie,*
> *I'll take mine.*

When Patricia cries,
you sit beside her,
pat her hand.

They like having you here.
Your gentle spirit calms things.

You see me in the lobby
and your face erupts with joy.

Smiling, smiling, smiling,
you hug me,
and I wonder,
> *Could anyone else*
> *ever love me like this?*

Death Dream

When you collapsed in the traffic lane
of the medical center parking garage,
it didn't occur to me, until much later,
how eerily similar this scene
to that recurring dream I had as a child,
in which you were struck by a car,
and lay dying,
while I bent over you, crying.

This time,
no car.

Your heart gave out.

And you didn't die,
until three days later,
because I blew my breath
into your lungs,
and
for a while,
at least,
kept you alive.

Setting It Right

They misspelled your last name
on your gravestone.

Our brother chuckles, affectionately.
This is so symbolic of her life, he says,
maybe we should just leave it.

That's just the point, I say.
One extra chromosome
skewed everything
just a little bit off-plumb,
but this one thing,
they can set right.

And so they do:
PHYLLIS ELAINE BOLENDER
November 6, 1940–December 3, 2000

So Much Treading

No one can know,
or needs to know,
how in the course
of our long marriage
these safe paths formed.

We learned
to walk around
briars and bogs,
keep away from
edges of cliffs.

Along these paths
we carved
by so much treading,
lie bones
picked of contention.

More significant
are the monuments
we raised,
rough cast, yet beautiful,
sacrificial altars
built by raw hands
lifting stone upon stone.

Some, not knowing,
wonder how we,
so different from each other,
could travel so long together.

We can't tell you.
We only know that
time alone taught
which notes
sing well along the way.

No one knows,
or needs to know,
the words
to our own peculiar song.

September's Secret

We still talk of that September day,
when we drove the Cascade highway.

Red, green and gold foliage
covered the mountain sides.

The sky shone cloudless,
the tangy, temperate air sparkled.

At one especially beautiful place,
where the highway crossed the river,
you suggested we pull off-road,
walk to a secluded spot.

We found it less satisfying
than we'd imagined,
the ground hard and prickly,
the fear of being caught.

What made the time magic though,
was your tender,
spontaneous idea.

That's what we carried home.
That's what we remember.

It Was a Useful Thing to Do

Fifty years ago,
in the cool, June morning
of our wedding day,
you and I picked the fresh,
rain-misted flowers
for the church —
peonies, delphiniums,
snap-dragons, lilies.

Into a marriage blow many winds,
and what will bend will bend,
and what is brittle will break.

Who is to say that our storms
and dry-spells,
freezes and thaws
were not all useful?

I was eighteen,
you were twenty.

We have picked many
crimson roses from our garden.

Neither of us can say,
    *I have lived with the same
    person these fifty years.*

Crows Flying

Beyond the tall evergreen trees
that shelter the physical rehab center,
across the lavender sky,
toward the rosy glow in the west,
an endless stream of crows.

A wide swath,
in no obvious formation,
fly apart from each other,
maybe two coming together
for a beat, then separating.

Mostly they are silent,
a few select *caws*
from designated speakers.

Where did they originate?

Where are they going?

A secret society
parallel to our own,
always there,
but largely unseen,
their presence now comforts me.

I prepare to drive home,
leaving my husband behind
in the rehab center,
crows still flying overhead,
an endless stream.

A Love Poem to My Husband on His Eightieth Birthday

Sometimes you are a rhinoceros,
ill-tempered and testy.

Sometimes you are a rock
holding your ground through my storms.

Sometimes you are the river that carries
our boat through perilous country.

Sometimes you are the steed
who rides me across the moors on your back.

Sometimes you are the frightened child
who needs me to rock you.

Always you are the loving embrace
that opens for me each night.

Post-Modern Goddess
To my granddaughter, Melissa

Like young Persephone,
innocence still clings
to your round cheeks.

You see world as new,
made just for your pleasure.

Like Athena,
you're Daddy's smart girl.

Your Master's degree completed,
you march toward your dreams,
most like Artemis,
restless for travel,
at home in Moscow or London,
fearlessly roaming the hills of Seattle.

Brown hair swings
over black leather jacket,
heel of your second-hand boot coming loose,
hole in the toe of your tights,
keys in hand as you stride the dark street.

Family Values

A civil war rages within the family.

Like Israel and Palestine,
both sides are right,
neither admitting error.

Try to stay neutral,
and you end up in the cross-fire.

The most innocuous word,
misspoken, sets them off,
a series of attack and retribution,
little chance of reconciliation.

Alliances deepen, divisions widen.

On Facebook's fertile battleground
the tension builds, the war plays out,
for all to see . . . until stony silence.

What would they lose
if they set aside their grievances?

What might they gain
by forgetting past hurts?

If we can't find forgiveness in the family,
how is there hope for the world?

Sixty-One Years of Marriage

He is what he is
and there's nothing
you can do about it.

You are what you are.

Two people entwined
like honeysuckle vines
begin to come apart
soon after the vows.

You had not bargained for this.

A drama progresses
without direction,
through happiness,
sorrow,
gain and loss,
hurt and forgiveness,
doors closed, doors opened,
bittersweet endurance.

It isn't easy,
and you wonder,
What if I had left?

Too late now.

You've set aside
a whole lifetime
of expectations.

You've grown
too loyal to each other,
fit into each other's groove.

Only death can sever
the golden bond
that holds you.

Conversation

Everything that needs to be said has already been said.
But since no one was listening, everything must be said again.
Andre Gide

At the mall, a couple sit
at a table outside Starbucks—
a man and a woman,
maybe in their fifties.

She leans forward a little,
elbows on table,
face alive with pleasure
of her subject.

He inclines his head toward her,
as if to catch every word.

He listens *not* as if he is thinking
of the next thing to say.

He listens as if he finds
every word she utters
utterly fascinating.

If only I could see myself
reflected in his eyes,
I would know
how to speak from my core.

I would never have need
to repeat myself,
him having heard me
so well the first time.

Roof

We both face that one hard fact —
one of us will die first,
my love,
statistically speaking,
probably you.

Always so practical,
you prepare for the day.

> *That roof*
> *should take care of you*
> *the rest of your life,*

you say, after the last nail is pounded
and the roofers drive away.

To hold you,
I'll think of something else.

Replace the dripping faucet in the bathroom.

We could use new vinyl in the kitchen.

Who will put my eye drops in at bedtime?

III

Wake to December

I Wake to December

Through a network of bare limbs,
a shell-pink glow
tints strings of clouds
that span the sky.

Foghorns sound mournful
warnings from the bay.

Stalks of summer annuals have browned,
and fallen leaves are swept
from streets and yards.

It's a slow time,
as autumn transitions into winter.

Only one-twelfth of the year remains,
and soon I will be eighty.

If only this body will keep on moving.
If only this mind will keep on thinking.
Days rush past and I'm not done.

Let me travel aware
of present wonders,
leaving behind a forgiven past,
looking not fearfully ahead.

I'll ignore the alarm bells
sounding everywhere

that ring for the young
with so much to lose.

I'll part with heavy possessions,
march into my winter season,
summer's warmth
still within my heart.

Trees in Love

Sun-drunk,
they shake their leaves,
dance with the April breeze.

Cones of fir and pine,
blossoms of apple and pear,
open wide to morning's rays.

Fecundity penetrates the air,
clings yellow mist to windshields,
swirls in paisley patterns on patios,
torments sinuses of the allergy-prone.

Take an antihistamine.

Go inside and close the windows.

Trees deserve their season of bliss.

Ubiquitous Crows

On *NPR*, the newsman says
not to fear the West Nile virus.
Just one percent of humans infected
experience serious symptoms.

When we begin to see dead crows,
he says, we'll know the disease
has reached our area.

In the *Washington Post*
an artist who lives in D.C. writes
that crows on her block,
even the family that nested in the tree
outside her window, are gone.

She can't recall precisely
when they disappeared.
Just empty skies
instead of blue-black silhouettes,
silence instead of raucous cries.

Here, in the Northwest,
from the pine tree
in my neighbor's yard,
I hear comforting caws.

Inky shapes punctuate
the landscape like characters
on rice paper paintings.

In the slant light of this late afternoon,
the last leaves on a birch tree

blaze like drops of sun from tips
of delicate branches.

Herds of ruddy sheep graze across
the threshold of the sky's purple pastures,
and a murder of crows flies overhead,
to roost in the tall firs
at the edge of my neighborhood.

Affliction

Are you my enemy or my friend?

You set boundaries to keep me in my place,
yet challenge me to claim my destiny.

Constrained by your defining terms,
boundaries you've set to keep me in my place,

I'll wrestle with you for my right to be
uncontained by your defining terms.

I challenge you and claim my destiny.

I'll wrestle you until I come to be
your limping enemy, your victorious friend.

So Many

So many seeds squandered,
    thrown where only sorrows grow,
        wrested in desolate darkness.

So many grown in fertile soil,
    fostering a tangled garden
        of abundance.

 So many things lost: children's young years
    slipping through my arms
        as in a dream.

So many braver colors
    I could have used to paint my past,
        finer wines to fill my glass.

So many ways I now reach out
    to grasp each new day's offerings,
        as gift and recompense for loss.

At First, She Never Asked

She saw scarcity
and feared refusal.

She learned to do with little.

Then she learned to ask
and found that refusal
didn't always follow.

She saw there was enough
for her, but wanted more.

Then she learned if she went after
what she wanted,
she didn't need to ask.

What power!

Then, she learned to answer,
to give without being asked.

Tahoma

Emblem of our higher selves,
you hover in the blue air,
shrouded in a robe of purest white.

We perceive you as immutable,
yet know your capricious nature.
On any given day,
your countenance could shatter,
a crystal goblet
blasted apart by fire from below.

A muck of melted ice
and powdered rock
would flow,
engulfing towns
and everything in your path.

Lulled by your calm beauty,
confident in our escape routes,
we go about our lives,
convinced that every day is safe,
disaster, a lifetime away.

Grief makes a sharp sound

like a knife slashing through my life,
separating what was from what is.

Grief sounds like *cancer,*
pain, death.

Grief doesn't let me forget,
if you go,

grief will stay here with me,
in the silence,

after.

This Cannot Be

My son is dying and I sit
in my favorite chair,
drink coffee,
plan my day,
check my phone,
watch birds fly
in and out
of the budding pear tree.

This can't be.
I should cry,
raise my voice in a howl,
crumple like a discarded love letter.

A new strength courses my blood.
A new resolve grips me,
pushes me out of bed in the morning,
makes me brush my teeth as always.

The sun comes up with its usual flame,
sinks down at its appointed time.
How can this be?

Consultation

I sit in my pastor's office seeking answers.
Are there certain things I should do,
or say, or feel?
I move about my day
in the usual way,
baffled
by the intrusive question,
>*How are you doing?*

I am the same.

Except for this new space I hold,
internal coldness that freezes,
prevents my tears.

My pastor gives me words meant
to take away anxiety and guilt.

>*Everyone deals with this in their own way.*
>*Ask your son what he needs.*
>*Be there for him as you find him.*
>*If he needs to talk, listen.*
>*If he needs you to talk, talk.*
>*If he wants you to silently watch*
>*the fishing channel with him, watch.*

I drive home somewhat reassured,
lie down to take a nap,
a newfound way
to help me through
these uncertain days.

After all, this day,
he still lives.

Self-Help for How to Grieve

My daughter tells me it's all right to cry.
I don't need to play the role of super-woman.

> *It's not as if he has a cold that can be cured.*
> *He's dying. It's okay to be broken.*

My friend tells me to scream and rail
to the gods at the unfairness of life.

> *Don't let them get away with this.*

I would cry, if I could.
I would scream and rail,
if I thought it would do any good.

I don't feel like a super-woman.
I'm helpless and confused.
What is a mother to do?

Another person tells me *Don't hover.*

> I need to hover.

Is there a manual with protocol and rules
for how to lose a son?
If so, give it to me, quick.
I need help.

Chemo

The March sky is unpredictable—
one minute, heavy gun-metal gray,
the next, white clouds scud across blue,
the sun bursts through.

This morning, my son begins
a five-hour drip,
poison combating poison,
venomous army facing off
against vicious foe,
scorched-earth strategy—no winners.

Three days of quarantine will keep me away.
Every two weeks, the same routine
until it stops—victory declared.

Or will the dread sky take over
and crush me with its sodden weight?

On the other side of my neighbor's fence,
the pear tree stands prepared
to fling its white blossoms open,
maybe by Wednesday.

The weatherman predicts
the sun will shine that day.

Chemo II

And so it begins,
his body shaken with sickness
greater than we had imagined.
I stand by, helpless and afraid.

This valley of the shadow of death
that I said I would not fear,
afflicts my soul with doubt,
takes away my defenses,
fills me with despair.

Trembling, I call my son,
praying he won't turn me away,
say he's too sick to see me.

He feels better, today,
happy to see me,
eats a little of the chicken soup
I brought him.

The sun shines again.
I drive home feeling useful,
hope restored,
until the next visit.

Chemo III

Only three more days
to his second round of chemo,
and he's not ready.

My son's response: *Oh, crap!*
to my question: *How are you doing?*
shows he's in the anger stage of grief.

This stuff changes your brain, he says.
It's making me mean.

He's thinking about quitting.
Why spend the last of his days like this?

Then he says he might give it one more try.

I tell him I will support his decision
either way, and he is grateful.

I hang up the phone,
feeling guilty and weak.

Tomorrow is Easter.
It will be sunny.

Why didn't I tell him to fight?

Night Petition

God, take into your care
these worrisome thoughts
keeping me awake.

If I lie here all night,
my eyes searching the darkness,
I'll be no good, come morning.

Neither profound nor righteous,
not worthy of becoming a poem,
these worries have no use.

I offer them only in hope
you will contain them,
keep them from flying off
in dangerous directions,
taunting me with dark imaginings.

A Mother's Goodbye

in memory of Galen Earl Cook
May 20, 1955–March 31, 2016

That day I brought you home,
your hungry cry filled me with fear.

We both launched into new life.
A girl of nineteen,
how could I meet your needs?

I watched in wonder as the flesh
on your skinny, newborn legs
blossomed and creased with fat
from my own body.

I marveled at each new expression
of your face,
movement of your hands.

When you began to crawl,
the toys I bought you lay unused,
as you pulled pots and pans
from my stove drawer
with a satisfying clang and bang.

A mother can never fully know
the mind of her son.
Some masculine part of him
stays hidden.
He listens to her motherly wisdom,
then goes off to pursue
his own adventures.

It was years before you told me
of the hang glider
you and your nerdy friend, Dan,
made from odds and ends and duct tape.

How you flew it on its virgin flight,
off a cliff, soaring above Maple Valley,
hundreds of yards below.

A mother can only pray,
as her son grows away from her,
as he must, to make his own
triumphs and mistakes.

From reckless youth,
to man, husband, father,
you followed your own quiet way.

Tank commander, electro-mechanic,
builder, gardener, tent-maker,
you shaped your world with skill.

You shied away from
my "by-the-numbers" religion.
The wilderness was your church.

You crafted your own tent and sleep-sack,
prepared survival food, and struck out,
into the woods, seeking solitude.

Your kind soul had a wild side —
a panther with a purr.

And you loved your dogs,
as they loved you.

I see I worried about all the wrong things.

No outside catastrophe struck you down.
Instead, an insidious monster attacked you
from the inside.

With no defense against it,
you escaped, slipped away,
with your usual aplomb.

And now you soar.
Goodbye, my son.
Be at peace.

Afterlife

It's your birthday,
and you're not here
to celebrate,
except, I feel your presence
as if you were.

After you died, I built
this special room
within my heart
where you and I can talk
as we never could before,
because, now we understand.

How can I, who finds it hard
to sustain belief in the afterlife,
converse so freely with you?

I tell no one.
I don't want to be told
all this is only fantasy
to console my grief.

If these pleasant talks with you
are mere illusions
to fill my longings,
they are no less
a medicine for my soul.

After you're gone,

rain waters the earth,
softens the soil.

The sky can cry,
why can't I?

New leaves grow
toward the sun.

The sky can cry,
why can't I?

My heart is thirsty desert.
Sorrow blows like wind.
No relief softens my pain.

The sky can cry,
why can't I?

Rain. So much rain.

Tide Interrupted

On the second birthday after my son's death

I'm sorry I cried
so little over you.
An Aquarius, I learned,
too well,
how to move my grief
aside for better times.

I fill my days in countless ways,
take my solitude in sips,
avoid empty spaces.

> With heavy stones
> I built a levy
> to keep at bay the pressing tide
> of stormy waves
> whose undulations
> would seize and set
> adrift my fragile craft.

I've much to do.
People depend on me.
I need to stay within an anchorage
safe from high tides
and low tides
and misplaced buoy markers.

One day you'll guide me
with word, or smell, or memory,
out beyond the reef,
where

risking the depths,
searching for a chest
full of precious tears,

I'll descend below the surface
to find what lies buried there.

Trilliums

Don't pick the trilliums
or they won't bloom for seven years.

I was a child,
and whether that was fact
or fiction,
I picked them.

Three white petals smiled
atop three heart-shaped leaves.

I shoved their straight stems into a fruit jar.

Wild heralds of spring,
if I didn't pick them,
their petals turned a sad purple,
then wilted away.

The more I picked,
the more they came back,
every year,
under the hemlock and maples.

I live now in Montana,
where trilliums
bloom under the trees
in my natural yard.

Myth of scarcity
has entered my old bones.

I don't pick the trilliums.

After Separation

Beneath my pear tree lies
a litter of cut branches —
growth that used to shield
its inner parts from sunlight.

Come the urgent flux of spring,
blind roots strive to sustain
what is no longer there.

In a surge toward survival,
the tree grows a little crazy,
sprouts a frenzy of useless shoots.

These too must be pruned,
for a season or two,
until the tree learns to thrive
without its severed parts.

Hymn of Thanksgiving

I pause my weeding
to listen to enchanting song
pour from an invisible bird
across the street in a tree.

To whom does it sing, and why?

The notes spill out with ease.

Perhaps he gives thanks
for his mate and the clutch
of eggs under her wings.

Perhaps he sings from a blissful breast,
not even aware he brings joy
to those who listen.

Starlings

The pine tree trembles
with the sound
of a thousand steely voices.

Amid the long needles,
I cannot see a single chorister,

though, some have flown
from the green sanctuary to rest
upon a power line,
like beads on a rosary.

Five thousand volts flow
beneath their unknowing,
ungrounded feet,
and not one feather singed.

I know a greater power pulsates
within my equivocal grasp.

If I should allow myself to leave
the crowded sanctuary,
dare to be aware,
ground myself to the source of light,
would I become serenely one
with its benevolent flow,
or would I burn
with its holy,
unquenchable fire?

As one,
the starlings rise in the air,
leave behind the tree, the wire,

and turn and dive
and write across the sky:
 Burn.
 Flow.

Star Song

Astronomers tell us that stars
    vibrate at frequencies corresponding
        to notes in musical scales.

And that vast strings of matter,
    thinner than an atom,
        stretch across space.

Strings on which the stars'
    vibrations strum celestial cords
        to play creation's symphony.

O, little race,
    existing on your little planet,
        your puny racket blocks

the heavenly harmony,
    as a thumb held close
        to an eye eclipses the sun.

Something far greater
    than you conducts
        this sublime orchestra.

Celestial music vibrates
    in every atom of the universe.
        Listen to its holy silence.

Useful Mistake

At a poetry reading about death,
one poet stands up to read.

Oops!
Instead of a poem,
she holds in her hand
the Google directions
on how to get there.

Privilege

As I write this poem,
machines in my home launder my clothes.

I don't need to cart them to a Laundromat,
and back, spend thirty bucks in coin.

Machines in my home launder my clothes,
using clean water piped into my house.

I don't lug water for miles in a jug,
or scrub my clothes in a pail.

Machines in my home launder my clothes,
as I write this poem.

To Denise Levertov, 1923–1997

I

Your letter advised,
don't *try* to write a poem,
wait and be ready.

Yet, you put your whole self
into forming yours.
No line-break or punctuation,
no "rhyme, chime, echo, repetition,"
escaped your careful craft.

Whether ant, bird or shadow,
moon, cloud or mountain,
myth or memory,
you used what you found
as *tesserae*
in your mosaic of metaphor.

You farmed your poems,
organically,
planting seeds of language
in rich alluvial soil,
harvesting their abundance
in the ripeness of time.

II

You traveled wide,
your "head a camera,"
your ears attuned
to the world's truth.

You flew to Viet Nam
(It was forbidden.)
to know who
we were bombing,
to know their faces,
their rice paddies,
their gentle way of living.
They shared their meals
when they learned
you had come in peace.
Back home, following news
of continuing carnage,
your first-hand knowledge —
missing limbs,
shattered eyes,
burned flesh —
left you open
to a bruised heart.

Meanwhile, angry Americans
lit a match
to your poems of witness.
Mercifully,
you died before 9/11
and the two useless wars
that it spawned.
How cruel it would have been
to put you through
all that, again.

Be at rest, dear prophet.
You gave it all you could.

Each new generation
must learn for itself
how to love.

End of War?

I asked my tai chi teacher,
*What if my opponent also knows
all the tai chi moves?*

He said, *If your opponent
also knows all the tai chi moves,
he will probably just go home.*

If all the army commanders of the world
taught their soldiers all the tai chi moves,
would they all just go home?

Home to loved ones who wait?
Home to dreams interrupted?
Home to sit down at table and eat?

New Friend

At the art museum,
two hours spent filling
my eyes with imagery,
I become aware
of your insistent presence.
My right hand,
resting in the crook of my left arm,
begins to tremble.
My gait concedes
to a slight unsteadiness.

For now, I shall call you P.D.
Soon, I'll be ready
to say your full name.

I have decided to love you,
a part of me I didn't ask for,
but won't reject,
now that I know you're not leaving.

You even serve a purpose,
sending me places I may otherwise
be too lazy to go,
if I didn't feel your tug.

Last week, I walked along Ruston Way,
felt the cool breeze coming off
the water on a hot afternoon.

Wednesday, I met a friend for lunch.

Today, I'm here.

You'll be my incentive
to fill my days
with nourishing pursuits,
reminding me,
that each moment I'm alive,
I can choose to be grateful.

Meditation on Michael Kenna's Photography

as seen at Tacoma Art Museum

A tree,
shaped by climbing children,
stands alone
in untouched expanse of snow.

Bony frames of a seaweed farm
reflect in quiet water.

Fences spaced up a snow-bound hillside,
lines of music on a white page.

Light, sky, and the silhouettes of trees
infuse towers
at a nuclear plant
with fragile beauty.

At the Catalan Masters Exhibit

Dali, Picasso, Mir, Miro—
an essence pervades the air
so distilled from the nature of things,
it stings the surface of my skin.

Beside me, you judge
with critical eye
whether each piece
does or does not
"do anything" for you.

As for me,
skin exfoliated by art,
pores exposed,
rare radiance
penetrates to my core.

Elegy for a Shepherdess

From *La Gardeuse de Moutons,*
painted by William-Adolphe Bouguereau, 1881

How lovely the scene behind you,
for which you show no interest.

Cliffs rise above pasture
where sheep graze.
Reddening shrubs, a river,
black hills in the distance.

What has harmed you,
shepherd girl,
that the quiet oval of your face
reflects the storm clouds
threatening to swallow the day?

You sit on a stone,
in homespun blues and grays.
Golden curls escape their scarf,
fall onto slumped shoulders.

A large button fastens a vest
over still unblossomed breasts.
Below your skirt, shapely legs
and bare feet cross at the ankle.

In one hand, an unfinished sock
and knitting needles.
In your lap, a switch for nicking
heels of wayward lambs.

Why are your lips so firmly set?

Gray eyes, too knowing for your age
look straight into mine.
I think you would tell me something,
if only you could trust.

Bonsai

For years, he treks through woods, scales shore cliffs, climbs mountain rocks, searching for a tree. Not one to which life has been kind — hearty branches climbing a straight trunk, in triumph to the sky. No. Instead, one grasping life by gnarly threads — twisted, bent, stunted by the elements. He takes great pains to move it, so not to break its tenuous hold on life so rare and ancient. As he plants it in its pot, he whispers, *I'll shape you.*

Year upon year, he trains its growth, splashes its thirst, listens to its silence.

Heaven and Earth
and Man between —
all One.

Four Friends

Every Thursday morning,
one married Methodist,
two widows —
Episcopal, Assembly of God —
and one iconoclastic Catholic nun,
hike the forest trails at Point Defiance Park.

This day,
they swish through layers of gold
and russet maple leaves,
pause to glean handfuls
of tangy, black huckleberries.

They talk of a daughter's wedding,
a book by Doris Lessing,
a retreat to the Palisades,
a friend who is dying.

Lingering fog turns sunlight,
filtering through firs and hemlocks,
into ethereal rays that stream
across their path.

Spider webs everywhere
shimmer with dew.

The trail skirts a cliff,
and the women stand silent,
looking across Commencement Bay.

From the indigo-blue water,
rises a silver cloud of terns.

Forming the tip of a pen,
they swoop and dive in graceful cursive script.

One woman turns to go.
The rest follow.

Such moments cannot be captured,
any more than fog
can hold onto sun-rays,
or words sea birds write in air
can tell a story,
or that these web-lined paths
will one day remember
the four friends who walked them.

Shrine

September morning,
walking through the woods
I come upon a large, granite rock,
speckled gray and black,
along the path.

Someone, or more than one,
has turned it into a shrine,
arranging pebbles
and a piece of green glass
on its smooth, inclined surface.

I add a tan, oval stone.
Embedded, white lines,
like petroglyphs,
tell its story.

It fits, and shifts
the restrained aesthetics
of the whole,
making it more beautiful.

If we could treat
our earth like this,
each person leaving behind
treasure thoughtfully placed,
all that is right will be left,
and all that is left will be right.

Curiosity, That's My Religion

Search and you will find,
said the one I trust as teacher.

Only yesterday, I saw
the irony in the prayer he taught us.

Forgive us . . . as we also have forgiven.
If I truly mean that, I'm in trouble.

Even as I say this prayer,
my mind dodges these words.

I'm dying to see what happens
when I die.

Is it the end of things,
or the beginning?

Don't tell me.

If you have it figured out,
you'll spoil the surprise.

When I Fly

I meet you in my quiet place.
I come with noisy, troubled mind.

You comfort my confusion and distress.
Bear me up as I grow weary.

Still the noisy static of my mind.

Where will I go when I fly from this body,
after it has grown too weary?

Comfort my confusion and distress.

Say that when I fly from this old body,
you'll meet me in a quiet place.

Invisible

December morning, six a.m.,
soft blue sky of emerging dawn,
empty of all but the radiant bodies
of Venus and the crescent moon.

Half-an-hour later,
both planet and satellite
are gone from sight,
enveloped in the sun's
dominant light.

Yet, I know for fact,
that both remain,
solid as a book
or this body.

Acknowledgments

The poet thanks the following publications in which her poems appeared, sometimes in previous versions:

Journals
Avalon Review: "Roof"

crosscurrents review: "Word Keeper"

Kaleidoscope: "Fierce Love," "Lady of the Manor"

Poet's West Literary Journal: "The Top Bunk," "They Used to Be My Toys," "Ubiquitous Crows," "Urban Capitalists"

Raven Chronicles: "At the Catalan Masters Exhibit," "Crustaceans," "Easter Egg Hunt," "The Peeler"

Spindrift: "Easter Egg Hunt"

Trillium: "Bonsai"

Websites
A Quiet Courage: "Phyllis's Fate"

Quill and Parchment: "To Denise Levertov"

Anthologies
Poetic Reflections–Creekside Anthology: "A Man Plans Differently," "Elegy for a Shepherdess," "Post Modern Goddess," "So Much Treading"

Kind of a Hurricane Anthologies:
   Secrets and Dreams: "Two Dreams"; *Shattered:* "Tahoma"; *Emergence:* "I Wake to December"; *Pyrokinection:* "Stepping Stone"

Women Writing: On the Edge of Dark and Light: "So Many," "New Friend"

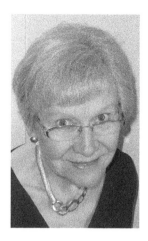

About the Author

Glenna Cook grew up in Olympia, Washington, where she married her husband, Kenneth, at age 18. They had three children (The oldest, a son, died of cancer in 2016.), and have nine grandchildren, and eight great-grandchildren. In 1990, she retired as training manager at U.S. West Communications, after twenty-five years of service, then immediately enrolled in college. She graduated from University of Puget Sound, Magna cum Laude, at age fifty-eight, with a B.A. degree in English Literature. While at U.P.S., she won the Hearst Essay Prize for the Humanities, and the Nixeon Civille Handy Prize for Poetry. She is a member of Phi Kappa Phi.

Her dream was to be a prose writer, but discovered a love for poetry at U.P.S., and after she graduated, and found herself the caretaker of both her mother and her sister, it fit well into the cracks of her time She has read her poetry in the Puget Sound region, and has published several dozen poems in journals and anthologies, such as *Raven Chronicles, Spindrift, crosscurrent review, Avalon Review,* and *Quill and Parchment*. In 2014, she was granted a residency at Hedgebrook, where she wrote some of the poems for this book.

Glenna has Parkinson's Disease, which she keeps at bay with medicine and a regular discipline of tai chi, yoga, and cycling exercises at the Y.M.C.A. She reads a lot, and enjoys playing the violin. Born in 1936, part of the "between" generation, who tends to see both sides, she is a Christian who feels kinship with other religions, a pacifist with sympathies for those who go to war, a feminist who loves men, and an environmentalist, pure and simple.

CPSIA information can be obtained
at www.ICGtesting.com
Printed in the USA
BVHW031043110219
539954BV00013B/1454/P